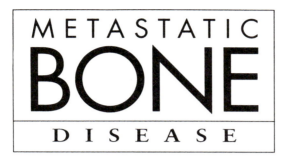

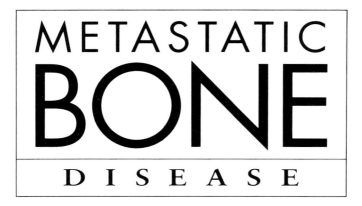

METASTATIC BONE DISEASE

EDITED BY R. COLEMAN & R.D. RUBENS

The Parthenon Publishing Group
International Publishers in Medicine, Science & Technology

Casterton Hall, Carnforth,
Lancs, LA6 2LA, UK

120 Mill Road, Park Ridge,
New Jersey, USA

Presentations to a scientific review meeting sponsored by
Ciba-Geigy held at the
Science Museum, London, 15 November 1991

Published in the UK and Europe by
The Parthenon Publishing Group Ltd.
Casterton Hall
Carnforth, Lancs. LA6 2LA

Published in North America by
The Parthenon Publishing Group Inc.
120 Mill Road
Park Ridge
New Jersey, NJ, USA

Copyright © 1992 The Parthenon Publishing Group Ltd.
ISBN: 1-85070-441-4

Typeset by AMA Graphics Ltd., Preston, Lancashire
Printed and bound in Great Britain by
Redwood Press Limited, Melksham, Wiltshire

Contents

List of participants

Chairmen

I. Boyle
University of Glasgow
Scotland
UK

R. D. Rubens
ICRF Clinical Oncology Unit
Guy's Hospital
London SE1 9RT
UK

Contributors

J.-J. Body
Department of Endocrinology
Institut Jules Bordet
Rue Héger-Bordet 1
B-1000 Brussels
Belgium

R. Coleman
YCRC Department of
    Clinical Oncology
Weston Park Hospital
Witham Road
Sheffield S10 2SJ
UK

D. Heath
Department of Medicine
Queen Elizabeth Hospital
Edgbaston
Birmingham B15 2TH
UK

A. Howell
Christie Hospital and Holt Radium
    Institute
Wilmslow Road
Withington
Manchester M20 9BS
UK

J. Kanis
Department of Human Metabolism
    and Clinical Biochemistry
Royal Hallamshire Hospital
Sheffield S10 2JF
UK

Preface

Bone metastases are common in breast and prostate cancer: over 70% of patients with advanced breast cancer have skeletal involvement. The morbidity caused by bone metastases – pain, hypercalcaemia, pathological fracture, neurological complications, bone marrow suppression – is both significant and long-lasting; if metastatic disease remains confined to the skeleton, survival can extend to a median of 24 months, with 20% of patients alive at 5 years. Such patients require skilled palliative and supportive therapy. In addition, hypercalcaemia itself, whether due to increased osteoclastic activity or enhanced renal retention of calcium, is associated with a number of unpleasant physical and psychological symptoms

Increasing recognition of the importance of osteoclast activation in mediating skeletal damage has led to the use of bisphosphonates – chemical analogues of pyrophosphate – in the treatment of both tumour-induced hypercalcaemia and osteolytic bone disease. This symposium, organised by Ciba-Geigy (Horsham, UK) and held in November 1991 at the Science Museum, London, discusses the biology and pathophysiology of bone metastases and the role of bisphosphonates in the treatment of tumour-induced hypercalcaemia and osteolytic bone disease, and includes a brief review of the non-oncological uses of bisphosphonates.

R. COLEMAN
R. D. RUBENS

1

Clinical aspects of metastatic bone disease

R. Coleman
YCRC Department of Clinical Oncology,
Weston Park Hospital, Sheffield, UK

SUMMARY

Bone metastases are of great clinical importance in patients with breast and prostate cancer, and cause considerable morbidity. This paper discusses the biology and pathophysiology of bone metastases, their imaging and assessment, and the available treatments. The increasingly important role of the bisphosphonates in the management of osteolytic bone metastases is emphasised.

INTRODUCTION

Bone metastases usually result in osteolytic lesions, with marked destruction of trabecular bone. Cortical bone is affected only relatively late in the process, but its involvement has profoundly adverse effects on bone structure.

Bone metastases are of particular clinical importance in patients with breast cancer, some 70–75% of whom develop bone metastases at some stage of their illness. Autopsy findings suggest that the figure may be even higher. Bone is also the commonest site of first distant recurrence (Table 1), and may be the only site of metastatic disease in about 20% of patients. Such cases have a long natural history, with a median survival of 2 years; 10% are still alive 5–10 years after first diagnosis of bone metastases, a fact that must be borne in mind when planning treatment.

Bone metastases can cause considerable morbidity. Pain is an almost invariable symptom requiring appropriate analgesia. About 15% of patients suffer a long-bone fracture, while many others have some degree

Table 1 Site of first recurrence in a series of 640 patients with breast cancer

Site of first recurrence	%
Local	38
Bone	29
Other soft tissue	12
Lung	7
Pleura	5
Liver	3
Brain	1
Other	5

of vertebral collapse. In addition, about 15–20% develop hypercalcaemia, with all its attendant symptoms and morbidity.

An interesting aspect of metastatic bone disease in both breast and prostate cancer is the phenomenon of osteotropism, the tendency of metastases to spread only to the skeleton. Many patients live through the entire course of advanced breast cancer with no evidence of metastatic spread outside the skeleton; in a series of 500 patients followed to death, almost 50% had disease clinically confined to the skeleton. The distribution of skeletal metastases tends to mirror the distribution of red bone marrow, being relatively common in the spine, ribs, pelvis and proximal appendicular skeleton and uncommon in the forearms, hands, feet, tibia, etc.

BIOLOGY AND PATHOPHYSIOLOGY OF BONE METASTASES

In health, the rates of bone resorption and formation are balanced and intimately related. Bone metabolism is controlled by two cells of different lineage: osteoblasts – concerned with bone formation – derived from the fibroblast system; and osteoclasts – involved in bone resorption – derived from the macrophage and monocyte system in the bone marrow. There is a complex and as yet poorly understood relationship between these two cells, known as coupling.

The metastatic process is a complex cascade of events (Figure 1). Circulating malignant cells enter the bone marrow space where they appear to be attracted to the endosteal (bone-forming) surface by

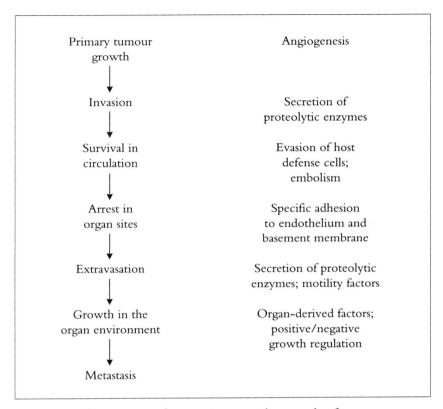

Figure 1   The sequence of metastasis, a complex cascade of events

chemotactic factors, probably collagen fragments. But the most important mechanism by which tumour cells cause bone destruction is the paracrine secretion of factors which stimulate osteoclasts to resorb bone (Figure 2). Many such factors have been suggested; in breast cancer, substances such as parathyroid hormone related protein (PTHrP), prostaglandins or cytokines may be involved.

Of secondary importance, and probably only relevant very late in the course of disease, is the ability of breast cancer cells to resorb bone directly through the production of proteolytic enzymes. The relative importance of this process is unclear, but it may account for some of the resistance seen to drugs that inhibit osteoclast function.

It is important to remember that tumour cells can also affect osteoblast function, which explains the sclerotic appearances sometimes seen on

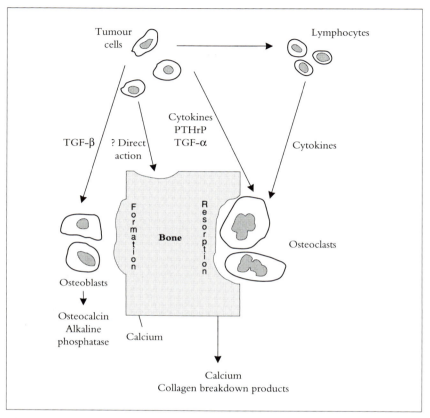

Figure 2 Mechanisms by which tumour cells may affect bone formation and destruction. TGF = transforming growth factor; PTHrP = parathyroid hormone related protein

X-ray. In most cancers there is both osteolysis and osteosclerosis, but in breast cancer osteolysis tends to predominate.

IMAGING AND ASSESSMENT OF BONE METASTASES

The bone scan

The methylene diphosphonate (MDP) bone scan, in which technetium-labelled diphosphonate is taken up preferentially at sites of increased osteoblast activity, can clearly demonstrate the multiple hot spots in the

Table 2 The influence of tumour size (T0–T4) on the outcome of bone scanning at presentation in 1155 women with breast cancer. (From Coleman et al 1988[1], with permission)

Tumour size	Number of patients	Positive baseline scan (%)	Bone relapse within 1 year (%)
T0	57	0	2 (4%)
T1	251	1 (0.3%)	3 (1%)
T2	582	17 (3%)	27 (5%)
T3	122	10 (8%)	11 (9%)
T4	143	19 (13%)	21 (15%)

femora, pelvis, spine or skull characteristic of advanced disease. But the number of patients with *early* operable breast cancer and a positive baseline bone scan is very small (Table 2), and it seems inappropriate to scan such patients routinely. Moreover, bone scanning is not a very specific tool for identifying metastatic disease; it will detect other skeletal pathology not due to metastatic disease, and may occasionally fail to identify lytic deposits clearly visible on X-ray (Figure 3). A bone scan will only show the presence of an osteoblastic response to a metastasis; occasionally in breast cancer, and more typically in multiple myeloma, this may be absent.

Computed tomography (CT)

In the patient presenting with a hot spot but with a normal X-ray, it may be appropriate to observe without further immediate investigations and/or treat on the basis of pain and the hot spot. However, to determine whether a hot spot is due to a metastasis requires targeted CT scanning (Figure 4).

Magnetic resonance imaging (MRI)

More sophisticated, and gradually becoming more widely available, is magnetic resonance imaging. This is now the modality of choice for investigating spinal cord compression, but is too expensive for routine assessment of bone metastases. Its use should be limited to the indication above, to research into specific lesions, for assessing the quality of response

15

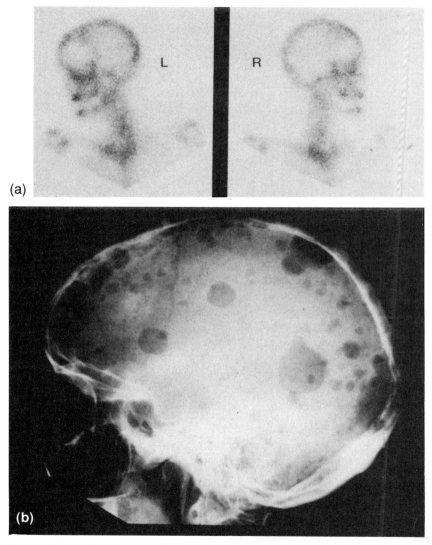

Figure 3　(a) Bone scans and (b) skull X-ray, the latter showing extensive lytic lesions not apparent on the bone scans

to different fractionation schedules of radiotherapy, and the effects of bisphosphonate therapy on individual lesions.

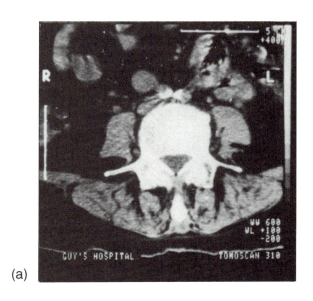

(a)

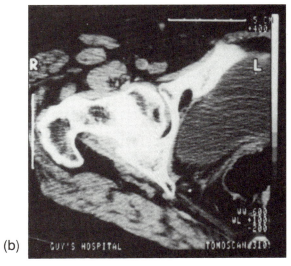

(b)

Figure 4 Computed tomographic (CT) scans of (a) spine and (b) femur in a patient with focal hot spots on the bone scan. Metastases were not visible on the plain radiographs but both lytic and sclerotic metastases are clearly demonstrated by CT

17

Assessing response to treatment

This is clearly of great importance, but extremely difficult (Table 3). Traditionally, doctors have relied on serial plain radiographs, but these can often be difficult to interpret (Figure 5). Assessment of symptoms is obviously vital, but there are very few validated techniques, especially in the important area of pain and mobility questionnaires. Alternative assessment methods such as tumour markers may be helpful in monitoring response, as may changes in bone metabolism, e.g. osteocalcin produced by osteoblasts.

Serial bone scans have been used to monitor progress, but can be misleading. A scan taken 3 months after baseline can appear much worse due to healing, the so-called flare response. Only 6–12 months after the introduction of systemic therapy can one realistically expect the bone scan to improve; it is of little value in the early assessment of response. Occasionally a CT scan is useful, particularly for sites that are difficult to see on plain X-ray (Figure 6).

Table 3   Methods of assessing response to treatment for bone metastases

Imaging
Plain radiographs
Computed tomographic scanning
Magnetic resonance imaging

Biochemical monitoring
Urinary calcium excretion
Urinary hydroxyproline excretion
Alkaline and acid phosphatase
Osteocalcin (Gla)
Serum calcium

Symptomatic assessment
Pain and mobility questionnaires
Analgesic requirements
Performance status

Tumour markers
CA15-3
CEA

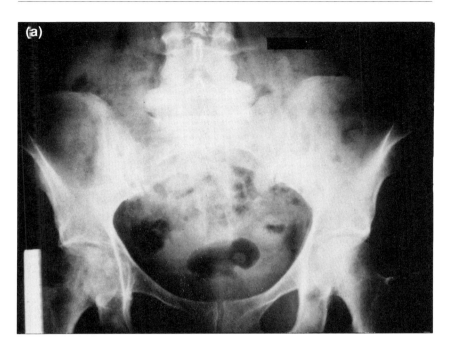

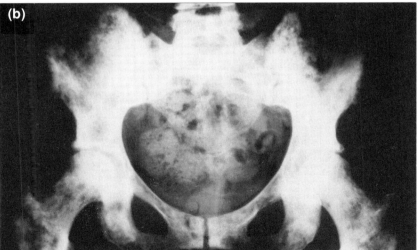

Figure 5 X-rays taken (a) before and (b) after systemic therapy with tamoxifen in a patient with multiple bone metastases. The X-ray in (a) shows multiple lytic lesions and a fracture: that in (b) (taken 6–9 months later) shows callus formation and sclerosis of lytic disease indicative of healing. The changes are often more difficult to interpret

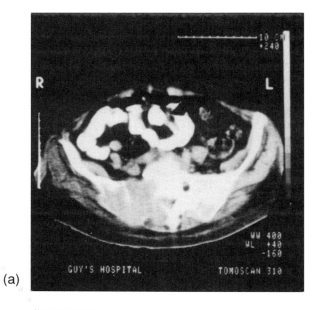

(a)

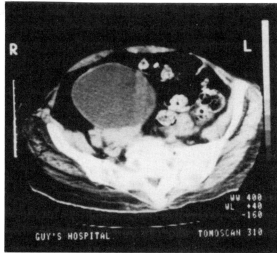

(b)

Figure 6 Computed tomographic (CT) scans taken (a) before and (b) after treatment with chemotherapy; (a) shows a large lytic lesion; (b) shows shrinkage of the tumour and reconstitution of the sacrum indicative of response to therapy

Table 4 Treatment options for bone metastases

Traditional treatments
Radiotherapy
Endocrine treatment
Chemotherapy
Orthopaedic intervention
Analgesia

New approach
Osteoclast inhibition

With respect to biochemical parameters, profound changes occur within a few weeks of starting successful systemic therapy. There is an increase in osteoblast activity, another manifestation of the healing response, coupled with a reduction in urinary calcium excretion. Urinary excretion of deoxypyridinoline can also be used as a marker of bone resorption. Biochemical monitoring has great potential; it is relatively inexpensive and reasonably quick. By combining biochemical parameters, an accurate prediction of response within a month of starting a new treatment is possible.

TREATMENT OF BONE METASTASES

The treatment options are listed in Table 4, divided into traditional treatments on the one hand and the relatively new concept of osteoclast inhibition on the other.

Traditional treatments

External beam radiotherapy

This remains the treatment of choice for a focal, painful metastasis. Simplified fractionation schedules can now provide good palliation with one, two or at most five fractions of radiotherapy; the prolonged schedules traditionally used are probably no longer necessary.

Targeted radiotherapy

This method, using radioisotopes which emit β-particles, is also effective in treating local disease. For example, [89]strontium, when injected intravenously, is taken up by areas of increased osteoblastic activity, emits β-particles and treats within a very short radius. This treatment has been used mainly in prostate cancer, which is usually more sclerotic than breast cancer. However, in a relatively small study[2] of strontium therapy in patients with metastases from breast cancer, about 20% achieved complete pain relief, another 20% had marked pain relief, 50% had moderate pain relief and only 10% had no pain relief. No patients in this study showed deterioration of symptoms. For multiple lesions, particularly when predominantly sclerotic, [89]strontium may be useful therapy. Its disadvantages are that it is difficult to give chemotherapy afterwards – due to bone marrow damage – and it is expensive.

Endocrine treatment

For the treatment of advanced breast cancer in premenopausal women this involves either some form of ovarian ablation – surgical or radiation-induced oophorectomy or a luteinising hormone-releasing hormone (LHRH) analogue – or tamoxifen. For postmenopausal women the main options are tamoxifen, progestogens or aromatase inhibitors.

Chemotherapy

There is no one chemotherapeutic regimen that is most appropriate. It must be remembered that patients have often had a significant amount of radiotherapy, so that the tolerance of their bone marrow is likely to be significantly reduced, from the radiotherapy itself and also from destruction of bone marrow by the tumour. Therefore, relatively non-myelosuppressive therapies or reduced doses of myelosuppressive drugs should be used.

Orthopaedic surgery

This has a role in the management of metastatic bone disease and should not be overlooked. Prophylactic fixation of impending fractures, spinal stabilisation to relieve pain due to instability, and prevention of spinal cord compression can benefit patients greatly. In addition, if fracture of a long bone occurs, the orthopaedic surgeon can restore mobility by internal fixation.

Bisphosphonates and osteoclast inhibition

Bisphosphonates have an important place in the treatment of osteolysis and bone metastases. They are a family of compounds, related to pyrophosphate, in which the oxygen of pyrophosphate has been replaced by a carbon atom (Figure 7); varying side-chains affect their activity against osteoclast function.

In normal health there is a close balance between resorption and formation (Figure 8). In metastatic bone disease, bone resorption is accelerated and, although some acceleration of bone formation occurs, the balance tips very much in favour of osteolysis, with loss of calcium

$$
\begin{array}{ccc}
& OH & OH \\
& | & | \\
O = P & - O - & P = O \\
& | & | \\
& OH & OH
\end{array}
$$
Pyrophosphate acid

$$
\begin{array}{ccc}
OH & CH_3 & OH \\
| & | & | \\
O = P - & C - & P = O \\
| & | & | \\
OH & OH & OH
\end{array}
$$
1-hydroxyethylidene-1, 1-
bisphosphonic acid (EHDP,
etidronate)

$$
\begin{array}{ccc}
OH & Cl & OH \\
| & | & | \\
O = P - & C - & P = O \\
| & | & | \\
OH & Cl & OH
\end{array}
$$
Dichloromethylidene
bisphosphonic acid (Cl$_2$MDP,
clodronate)

$$
\begin{array}{ccc}
& NH_2 & \\
& | & \\
& CH_2 & \\
& | & \\
OH & CH_2 & OH \\
| & | & | \\
O = P - & C - & P = O \\
| & | & | \\
OH & OH & OH
\end{array}
$$
(3-amino-1-hydroxy-
propylidene)-1, 1-
bisphosphonic acid (APD,
pamidronate)

Figure 7 The structure of pyrophosphate acid and the three most commonly used bisphosphonates – etidronate, clodronate and pamidronate

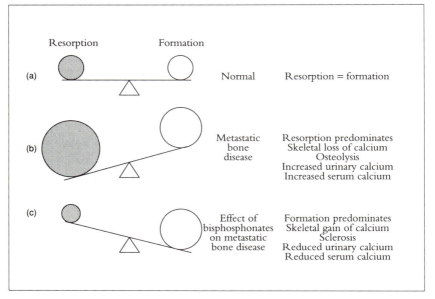

Figure 8 The close balance in health between bone resorption and formation (a) is tipped in favour of accelerated resorption by metastatic bone disease (b). Bisphosphonates inhibit bone resorption, with very little acute effect on the rate of bone formation (c)

from the skeleton and increased levels of calcium in the serum and urine. A bisphosphonate such as pamidronate inhibits bone resorption specifically, with very little acute effect on the rate of bone formation: calcium returns to the skeleton and urinary and serum calcium levels fall.

A single intravenous injection of pamidronate results in a marked reduction in urinary calcium excretion and, if the patient is hypercalcaemic, rapid control of hypercalcaemia. Pamidronate is long-acting, and can be given every 2, 3 or 4 weeks as long-term therapy for osteolysis.

CONCLUSIONS

Bisphosphonates are already established as the treatment of choice for hypercalcaemia, and provide useful palliative therapy for bone metastases. They also have potential uses in preventing metastatic involvement of bone and in protecting the normal skeleton against the unpleasant effects of castration performed by surgery, radiotherapy or chemotherapy. For the future, there is a continuing need for greater understanding of the mechanisms of osteolysis, of the factors that cause osteotropism, and of the role of bisphosphonates in the treatment and prevention of metastatic bone disease.

REFERENCES

1. Coleman, R. E., Fogelman, I. and Rubens, R. D. (1988) A reappraisal of the baseline bone scan in breast cancer. *J. Nucl. Med.*, **29**, 1354–9
2. Robinson, R. G., Blake, G. M., Preston, D. F., et al (1989) Strontium-89: treatment results and kinetics in patients with painful metastatic prostate and breast cancer in bone. *Radiographics*, **9**, 271–81

2

Bone biology and the role of bisphosphonates

J. Kanis, T. H. Taube, J. Aaron and M. N. C. Beneton
Department of Human Metabolism and Clinical Biochemistry,
Royal Hallamshire Hospital, Sheffield, UK

SUMMARY

Bone is a living tissue, the structure and function of which is perturbed by neoplastic infiltration, whether osteolytic or osteosclerotic. In health, bone remodelling maintains a balance between bone destruction and bone formation brought about by the unified action of osteoclasts and osteoblasts, the process of coupling. Neoplastic activation of the skeleton results in bone loss, whether by the creation of erosion cavities which are then filled incompletely by new bone, or by uncoupling the actions of osteoclasts and osteoblasts, leading to progressive erosion or inappropriate deposition of bone on quiescent surfaces or within the marrow cavity. Various systemic and local factors are involved in this process.

Bisphosphonates, stable chemical analogues of pyrophosphate, inhibit the osteoclast-mediated bone resorption associated with neoplastic activation, and are strongly adsorbed onto mineralised tissue. They may also inhibit the production of mature osteoclasts, and reduce their number to normal. In clinical trials bisphosphonates have been shown to be effective in the management of hypercalcaemia of malignancy (in conjunction with saline repletion), and to reduce the incidence of bone pain due to malignancy. There is more recent evidence that their long-term administration may alter the expression of tumour activity on bone cells and thus afford long-term protection to the skeleton.

INTRODUCTION

This paper reviews the biology of bone and the processes involved in neoplastic activation of the skeleton. Metastatic disease, whether osteo-lytic or osteosclerotic, affects skeletal tissue in several ways; to know how the skeleton responds and how it is perturbed in neoplastic disease requires a clear understanding of bone biology.

BIOLOGY OF BONE

Bone comprises mineralised tissue of two types: an inner core of *trabecular* or spongiform bone covered by an outer shell of *cortical* bone which is made more resistant to compressive and torsional forces by the intercon-necting lattice-work of trabecular bone within (Figure 1). The human skeleton is stronger *in vivo* than cast-iron is *in vitro*, due to its capacity to repair the fatigue damage that occurs in all solid structures, a process particularly prominent in trabecular bone. Although trabecular bone contains only 20–25% of total body calcium, it gives structural rigidity to

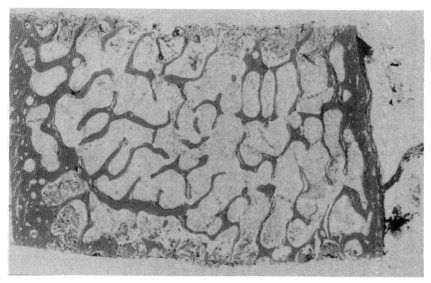

Figure 1   Section of bone, showing the compactness of cortical bone and the lattice-work structure of trabecular bone within

the skeleton, and lesions that occur in trabecular tissue have a significant impact on the ability of the skeleton to resist compressive and torsional forces.

Bone is a living tissue. Its life is regulated by the activity of bone cells on its surface. Because the surface-to-volume ratio of trabecular bone is much higher than in cortical bone, disease processes tend to occur sooner and more floridly in trabecular bone than at sites of cortical tissue. The vast majority of normal bone surfaces are covered by quiescent, inert lining cells but at specific loci there are congregations of active cells, either *osteoblasts* – responsible for the synthesis of an organic matrix and its mineralisation – or giant, multinucleated *osteoclasts* responsible for bone destruction.

The balance between bone destruction and formation is governed by the process of bone remodelling (Figure 2). Osteoclasts, attracted to a site of fatigue damage, remove the fatigued bone by creating an erosion cavity. Osteoblasts are then attracted to sites of prior resorption, a phenomenon called coupling, and thereafter synthesise the organic matrix which will eventually fill in the resorption cavity. This new wall of bone becomes fully mineralised to complete the process of remodelling. In health, some two million bone remodelling units are present at any one time, accounting for about 95% of skeletal turnover.

NEOPLASTIC ACTIVATION OF THE SKELETON

There are several mechanisms of bone loss in malignant disease. The first relates to the balance between formation and erosion of bone. Coupling is preserved, in the sense that osteoblasts are attracted to sites of previous resorption, but the amount of new bone formed is inadequate to balance that resorbed. This may be due to decreased functional competence of osteoblasts, to decreased numbers of osteoblasts, or to an increase in the activity or numbers of osteoclasts. Irrespective of the cause, for each remodelling sequence there is a small but finite amount of bone loss. In these circumstances, accelerating the rate of bone remodelling by increasing the number of bone remodelling units will merely amplify the rate of bone loss.

This process is common to many forms of neoplastic activation, and results in the diffuse osteoporosis seen in myelomatosis and in some

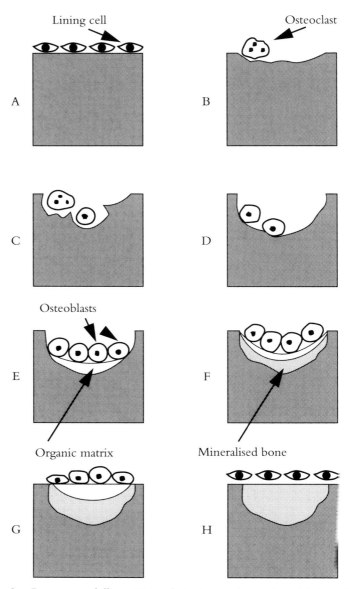

Figure 2 Bone remodelling. Osteoclasts attracted to a site of fatigue damage remove the fatigued bone and create an erosion cavity (B–C). Osteoblasts are attracted, and synthesise the organic matrix which will fill in the resorption cavity (D–F). The new bone eventually becomes fully mineralised to complete the remodelling process (G–H)

patients with breast cancer. Reduction in bone volume is associated with increased numbers of bone remodelling units: processes of resorption and formation have been amplified, but the amount of bone formed is less than adequate for the increased bone turnover.

Another mechanism of bone loss is uncoupling, which can produce holes in bone (Figure 3). In this situation, an erosion cavity fails to attract osteoblasts, the coupling signal having been lost. Progressive erosion may, in time, transect a trabecular structure. Even if osteoblasts are eventually attracted to sites of previous resorption, they are incapable of restoring the integrity of trabecular tissue. The disruption of the architecture and functional competence of affected tissue is disproportionate to the amount of bone lost.

Conversely, there can be a positive uncoupling, the deposition of bone not at sites of previous resorption but at quiescent surfaces, or condensation of stromal elements within the marrow to give rise to new bone formation. This latter is the characteristic mechanism of *osteosclerotic*

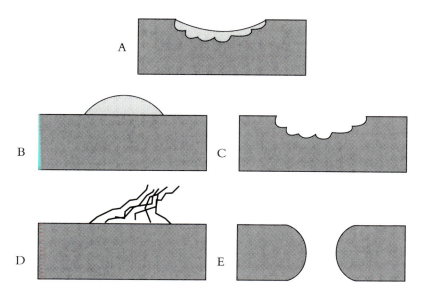

Figure 3 Mechanisms of bone loss or abnormal bone formation dependent on uncoupling between osteoblasts and osteoclasts. A = successive erosion without matching osteoblastic response; B = deposition of new bone on a quiescent surface; C = erosion with no osteoblastic response; D = new bone formation within the marrow cavity; E = transection of trabecular bone

Table 1 Systemic and local factors likely to be of variable importance in the neoplastic activation of osteoclasts

Systemic	Local
Parathyroid hormone related protein (PTHrP)	Lymphotoxin
Transforming growth factor α (TGF-α)	Prostaglandin E
Interleukin-1, interleukin-6	Procathepsin D
Tumour necrosis factor	
1,25 $(OH)_2$ cholecalciferol	
1,24 $(OH)_2$ cholecalciferol	

metastases, in which the normal trabecular architecture is overlaid by new bone deposited on quiescent surfaces. However, most of the skeletal morbidity associated with neoplastic disease arises from *osteolytic* metastases, in which trabecular bone is destroyed by a progressive wave of bone resorption in the complete absence of bone formation.

One of the cardinal features of metastatic bone disease, whether osteosclerotic or osteolytic, is that it is mediated by perturbation or activation of normal bone cells by both systemic and local factors (Table 1). Procathepsin D is likely to be important in some patients with breast cancer and focal skeletal disease. The interleukins and parathyroid hormone related protein (PTHrP) are potent activators of osteoclast-mediated bone resorption, and may account for generalised bone loss. The mechanisms vary in different patients, even in those with the same tumour type.

THE ROLE OF BISPHOSPHONATES

Bisphosphonates (Figure 4) are analogues of pyrophosphate, a natural substrate which inhibits bone resorption by reducing the number and activity of osteoclasts and probably also has a role in bone mineralisation. The rapid cleaving and enzymatic hydrolysis of pyrophosphate led to development of the carbon-substituted bisphosphonates which are resistant to such enzymatic hydrolysis. Like pyrophosphate, the bisphosphonates inhibit osteoclast-mediated bone resorption, and are also chelated and strongly adsorbed onto mineralised tissue. This property not only increases their therapeutic potential by delivering the drug to its site of action, but also reduces the potential for systemic toxicity at other sites.

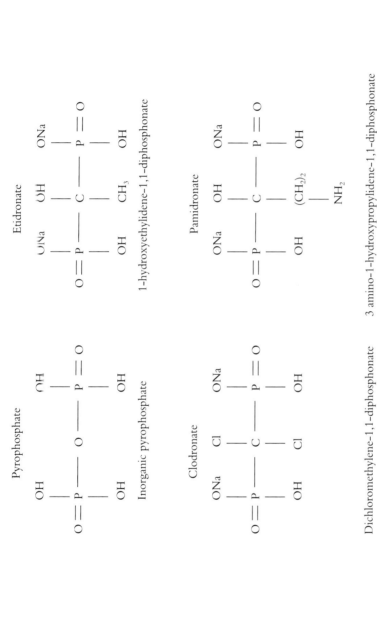

Pyrophosphate

Inorganic pyrophosphate

Etidronate

1-hydroxyethylidene-1,1-diphosphonate

Clodronate

Dichloromethylene-1,1-diphosphonate

Pamidronate

3 amino-1-hydroxypropylidene-1,1-diphosphonate

Figure 4 Structure of pyrophosphate and the three most commonly used bisphosphonates – etidronate, clodronate and pamidronate

33

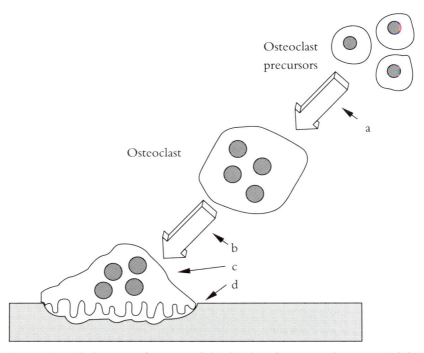

Figure 5 Likely sites of action of the bisphosphonates. They may inhibit accession of mononuclear osteoclast precursors to the multinucleated cell pool (a), or attachment of osteoclasts to the bone surface (b). Pretreating the bone surface with a bisphosphonate makes it unpleasant to the osteoclast, either disrupting its internal function (c) or preventing resorption of bone (d)

Bisphosphonates act by a variety of mechanisms (Figure 5). They are certainly adsorbed onto the bone surface (the basis of bone scanning), and there is good experimental evidence that pretreating the bone surface with a bisphosphonate makes it unpleasant to osteoclasts, either because they dislike the 'taste', or because the incorporation of the bisphosphonate into the osteoclast disrupts its function. On the other hand, there is also good evidence that some bisphosphonates inhibit both the attachment of osteoclasts to the bone surface and the accession of mononucleated osteoclast precursors to the multinucleated cell pool. It is probable that all the bisphosphonates act in all these various ways, but the relative importance of each action may be different. For example, after treatment with pamidronate, osteoclasts remain abundant in the marrow cavity but

Table 2   Percentage of patients either hypercalcaemic or hypocalcaemic by type of bone metastasis: osteoblastic, osteolytic or mixed. (From Kanis et al [1], with permission)

Bone metastasis type	Number of patients	Hypercalcaemic (%)	Hypocalcaemic (%)
Osteoblastic	59	0	25
Mixed	15	7	7
Osteolytic	60	28	3
Unknown	21	14	9

no longer resorb bone; with other bisphosphonates there is an absence of osteoclasts after prolonged treatment. These findings show that bisphosphonates are able to inhibit the osteoclasts associated with neoplastic activation, and to reduce osteoclast numbers to normal.

The morbidity associated with increased bone resorption is primarily of three kinds – hypercalcaemia, bone pain, and skeletal fracture, and it is osteolytic rather than osteoblastic metastases that are associated with this morbidity, particularly in the case of hypercalcaemia (Table 2).

In assessing the effects of bisphosphonates, it is important to understand that, even though the induction of hypercalcaemia may be related to increased resorption, it is often maintained by other factors, in particular extracellular volume depletion. The essential first step in the management of hypercalcaemia is therefore the restoration of extracellular volume by saline repletion. In the case of solid tumours, nothing is to be gained by the addition of corticosteroids. Some hypercalcaemic patients will not require additional treatment, provided they receive specific treatment for their cancer. In the clinical research setting, the best way to assess the effects of a bisphosphonate on serum calcium is to treat patients initially with saline until serum calcium is stable, and only thereafter give the bisphosphonate. This increases confidence that any subsequently observed changes are related to the bisphosphonate rather than to concurrent treatment. In addition, indirect indices of skeletal metabolism – reduction in serum calcium and decreased urinary excretion of calcium and hydroxyproline (in part derived from skeletal catabolism) – can be used to verify the inhibition of bone resorption.

Shortly after the introduction of bisphosphonates for the treatment of hypercalcaemia, it was noted that many patients experienced a reduction in bone pain. Studies were undertaken to determine whether this was a placebo effect, whether it was due to the reduction in serum calcium favourably affecting the pain threshold, or a specific action of the bisphosphonates. A recently published study[2], in which patients with bone pain were randomly allocated to receive a single intravenous infusion of clodronate or placebo, and then crossed over to the other treatment, showed that most patients (58%), and indeed most physicians (66%), preferred the active agent, suggesting that bisphosphonates are able, at least acutely, to reduce bone pain.

If bisphosphonates can inhibit osteoclasts and decrease the acute manifestations of increased bone resorption, might they also be able to alter the long-term expression of skeletal disease? It has recently become clear that, despite an apparently adequate response to specific therapy, progressive bone disease is characteristic of many tumours, and current methods of assessing bone response are totally inadequate for the identification of this in most cases. A recent Phase II study[3], in which patients received both chemotherapy and clodronate, has shown that the bisphosphonate can prevent or mask relapse – at least so far as the skeleton is concerned – raising the possibility that long-term administration of bisphosphonates may alter the expression of tumour activity on bone cells and therefore the natural history of osteolytic bone disease.

REFERENCES

1. Kanis, J. A., McCloskey, E. V., O'Rourke, N., et al (1991) Diphosphonates in hypercalcaemia and osteolytic bone disease. In Powles, T. J. and Smith, I. E. (eds.) *Medical Management of Breast Cancer*, pp.317–23. (London: Martin Dunitz)
2. Paterson, A. H. G., Ernst, D. S., Powles, T. J., et al (1991) Treatment of skeletal disease in breast cancer with clodronate. *Bone*, **12**, 525–30
3. McCloskey, E. V., Paterson, A. H. G., Powles, T. J., et al (1990) Clodronate decreases the incidence of hypercalcaemia and major vertebral fractures in metastatic breast cancer. *J. Bone Min. Res.*, **5** (Suppl. 2), 241 (Abstr.)

DISCUSSION

Dr R. Coleman (*Sheffield, UK*) Rehydration is essential in the treatment of hypercalcaemia of malignancy, but with both intravenous and oral bisphosphonates so readily available and easy to use, there is a danger that some doctors will move away from treating hypercalcaemia appropriately by rehydration with saline followed by bisphosphonate, and just use the bisphosphonate alone.

Dr B. M. J. Cantwell *(Newcastle, UK)*   In my experience it appears safe to treat moderate to severe hypercalcaemia associated with breast cancer by means of an intravenous infusion of bisphosphonate with immediate rehydration or followed directly by rehydration, but I do agree that rehydration is essential.

Professor Kanis   I believe that treatment should be given concurrently – by intravenous volume repletion, if necessary with a bisphosphonate to inhibit bone resorption. Some patients can tolerate stable hypercalcaemia for years, for example in primary hyperparathyroidism; this does not require emergency treatment, and can be managed on an outpatient basis if necessary. In contrast, the unbalanced and progressive hypercalcaemia seen in many forms of bone disease, but classically in the case of bone cancer, requires urgent treatment.

Dr I. Boyle *(Glasgow, UK)*   There was initially some concern about additional toxicological problems with intravenous bisphosphonates in very dehydrated patients, but this proved unfounded.

Dr Cantwell   I agree, but we always rehydrate patients immediately after administration of the bisphosphonate.

Dr Boyle   Professor Kanis, do you have any thoughts on the possible importance of physical stress in determining nidation of metastatic cells in the skeleton?

Professor Kanis   Normal stresses and strains induced in bone are very important in determining the balance between formation and resorption. Although I implied in a rather simplistic way that bone formation exactly matched bone resorption in each remodelling unit, that is clearly not the case, particularly in trabecular tissue, which exhibits local imbalances so that its architecture can respond adequately to the strains imposed. Whether these processes are affected by metastatic deposits is not known, although the pattern of metastases in immobilised patients seems to be the same as that in mobile patients.

3

Treatment of tumour-induced hypercalcaemia

J.-J. Body
Department of Internal Medicine and Endocrinology, Institut
Jules Bordet, Brussels, Belgium

SUMMARY

Traditional management of tumour-induced hypercalcaemia comprises specific antineoplastic therapy, intravenous rehydration, and inhibition of bone resorption with drugs such as calcitonin or mithramycin. Bisphosphonates are potent inhibitors of bone resorption, and are effective in reducing elevated serum calcium levels to normal and in reducing urinary excretion of calcium. The role of the bisphosphonate pamidronate (APD) in the management of tumour-induced hypercalcaemia is considered under various headings: the efficacy of single or daily infusions; the dose–response relationship; optimal therapeutic modality; overall efficacy; side-effects; need for combination with other drugs; and efficacy on second and subsequent courses of treatment. Pamidronate can normalise serum calcium in 90–95% of hypercalcaemic cancer patients at a dose of 1.0–1.5 mg/kg bodyweight, whether given as a single infusion or in divided doses over 2–3 days. Response to pamidronate at these dose levels is not influenced by tumour type or extent of bone metastases. The drug is well tolerated. Loss of efficiency in second and subsequent courses could be overcome by increasing the dose or by maintenance therapy with regular infusions or daily oral dosing.

INTRODUCTION

The traditional approach to the management of tumour-induced hypercalcaemia has three aspects: general measures, inhibition of bone resorption, and other miscellaneous treatments.

General measures involve specific antineoplastic therapy, intravenous rehydration with saline infusions, and avoiding immobilisation, thiazide diuretics and vitamin D.

The first essential therapeutic step is to administer a saline infusion to restore the circulating volume. This will improve the patient's clinical status, as most of the symptoms of hypercalcaemia are due to or increased by the reduced circulating volume. Such treatment usually has little effect on calcium levels, with a median decrease of about 1.0 mg/dl, according to a review of the available data.

Since the major pathology in tumour-induced hypercalcaemia is increased osteoclastic activity, it is also essential to inhibit bone resorption. *Calcitonin* is a natural antiosteoclastic hormone, the main advantages of which are rapid onset of action and negligible toxicity. However, its efficacy is variable, partial and transient; after a few days the calcium level starts to rise again even if the dose is increased. *Mithramycin* is another specific antiosteoclastic drug, but its efficacy is highly variable and it is toxic on repeated administration. Corticosteroids are only indicated for haematological malignancies, not for hypercalcaemia complicating solid tumours. The miscellaneous therapies are mostly outdated, but oral phosphorus can be useful in a few patients with chronic moderate hypercalcaemia, although its use is limited by digestive side-effects. Intravenous phosphorus has no place in therapy, due to the major risk of extraskeletal calcium precipitation.

THE ROLE OF BISPHOSPHONATES

There are several bisphosphonates available. *Etidronate* is almost always given at a dose of 7.5 mg/kg/day for 3 days, although some doctors continue for 7 or even 10 days. In a recently published study[1] with a large number of patients, 63% became normocalcaemic, but when calcium levels were corrected for hypoalbuminaemia the response rate fell to 24%. *Clodronate*, given variably at doses of 300–1000 mg/day for 1–10 days, is claimed to have an 80–90% success rate[2,3]. This is probably true if the drug is given for more than 1 day, but unlikely following a single-day infusion. In a recent trial[4] with *tiludronate*, given at doses from 3.0–6.0 mg/kg/day for 3 days, we obtained a success rate of 72%, but only 61% if the calcium levels were corrected for hypoalbuminaemia. The relatively high doses required involve a substantial risk of nephrotoxicity, and in my opinion this drug is not indicated for the treatment of tumour-induced hypercalcaemia. *Aminohexanebisphosphonate* (AHBP) has been in use for several years. In a recent trial[5] which gave a single infusion of 5 mg, seven out of nine patients became normocalcaemic by day 6.

THE PLACE OF PAMIDRONATE

The role of pamidronate in the management of tumour-induced hyper-calcaemia will be discussed under eight heads.

Efficacy of repeated daily infusions

Pamidronate was first given as daily 15 mg infusions over 2 hours until patients became normocalcaemic. In a multicentre trial[6], 90% of 132 hypercalcaemic cancer patients so treated became normocalcaemic within 3–4 days (median value). This fall was mirrored by a decline in the fasting urinary excretion of calcium, a sensitive and easily measured index of the rate of bone resorption.

As part of this trial[7], we successfully treated 24 patients, all of whom became normocalcaemic after a mean of three daily doses (Figure 1). The prolonged efficacy of pamidronate was demonstrated in 17 patients – three no longer under treatment, 14 with evident failure of further antineoplas-tic treatment – in whom serum calcium levels remained normal for a median of at least 3 weeks (range from > 1 to > 8 weeks), confirming prolonged efficacy of the drug.

Efficacy of a single infusion

This form of treatment was developed by Thiébaud and Burckhardt[8], who treated ten hypercalcaemic cancer patients by a single 24-hour infusion of 60 mg pamidronate, and showed that all became normocal-caemic.

Dose–response relationship

It can be difficult to know whether a dose–response relationship exists when dealing with efficient drugs. In a Phase I dose–response trial[9]

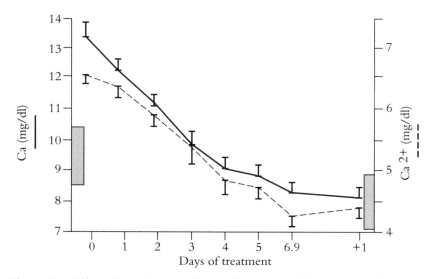

Figure 1 Effect of pamidronate 15 mg daily (given as 2-hour infusion) on total and ionised serum calcium levels in 24 and 14 patients, respectively, with tumour-induced hypercalcaemia (mean ± SEM). Hatched columns along y axes represent normal range. The lines on the graph show normalisation of serum calcium in all patients after a mean of three daily doses. From Body et al[7], with permission

performed several years ago, patients received one of six possible doses of pamidronate, starting at the very low dose of 0.01 mg/kg/day and rising to the very high dose of 3.0 mg/kg/day: all doses were given as 2-hourly infusions for 3 days. The two lowest doses were insufficient to achieve substantial falls in either serum or urinary calcium levels, but there were no significant differences in response between the other four doses (Figure 2). Similar dose–response relationships have been shown in patients ($n = 52$) receiving one of four doses of pamidronate (30, 45, 60 or 90 mg) as a single 24-hour infusion[10]. Only nine patients did not become normocalcaemic, eight of them in the low-dose groups receiving 30 or 45 mg.

Other groups have not found this dose–response relationship, probably due to the inclusion of too few patients, or of patients with only moderate hypercalcaemia, or to the prescription of insufficiently high doses or too short a follow-up period. Table 1 presents all the well-documented studies

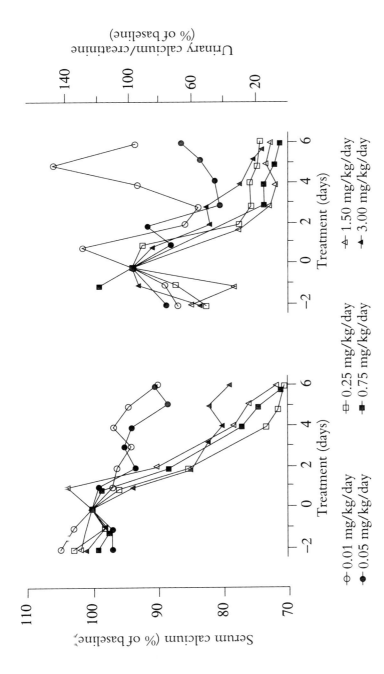

Figure 2 Effect of pamidronate given at six different doses for 3 days, each dose administered as a 2-hour infusion, on serum calcium and urinary calcium/creatinine levels in patients with tumour-induced hypercalcaemia. From Body et al[9], with permission

Table 1   Dose–response to pamidronate in tumour-induced hypercalcaemia – review of the literature. Compare data with Figure 3. (From Body[13])

Authors	Mean initial serum calcium (mmol/l)	Total dose of pamidronate (mg)	Number of patients	Normalisation of serum calcium (%)
Coleman and Rubens[14]	3.15‡	5–15	23	18 (78)
Ralston et al[15]	3.18	5–25	17	9 (53)
Cantwell and Harris[16]	3.35+	30	16	10 (63)
Body et al[11]	3.45	30★	11	8 (73)
Thiébaud et al[10]	3.28	30–45	26	18 (69)
Mannix et al[17]	3.58	45	25	18 (72)
Ralston et al[15]	3.15	45	19	16 (84)
Morton et al[18]	3.40+	60†	30	28 (93)
Sawyer et al[19]	3.33+	60★	23	21 (91)
Thiébaud et al[10]	3.60	60–90	26	25 (96)
Body et al[11]	3.40	90★	22	20 (91)
Body et al[7]	3.33‡	60–135†	24	24 (100)

★Dose calculated on weight basis; †administered over ≥ 2 days; ‡calcium concentrations not corrected for protein levels; +patients not previously rehydrated

of pamidronate in tumour-induced hypercalcaemia, the doses given in each, and the number and percentage of patients who became normocalcaemic after therapy. Plotting the percentage of patients achieving normocalcaemia against the total dose(s) received in each study gives a linear relationship ($r = 0.83$, Figure 3). To obtain a 90% success rate would require a dose of 80–90 mg, which is indeed our experience.

Optimum therapeutic modality

We undertook a randomised comparison[11] between a treatment consisting of daily infusions of pamidronate 0.5 mg/kg/day for 3 days and single infusions, either 1.5 mg/kg or 0.5 mg/kg (Figure 4). A dose of 1.5 mg/kg, given as a single infusion or divided into three daily infusions, was equally effective in reducing serum calcium levels and the urinary excretion of calcium.

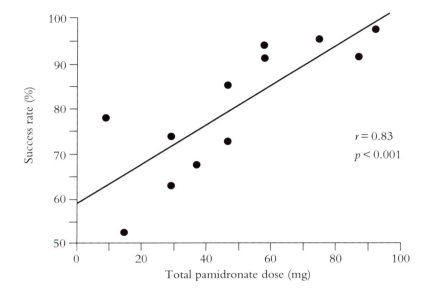

Figure 3 Dose–response effects of pamidronate in tumour-induced hypercalcaemia: the percentage of patients achieving normocalcaemia in each study detailed in Table 1 plotted against the dose of pamidronate used. From Body[13]

Overall efficacy of pamidronate

Do patients with humoral hypercalcaemia respond less well than those with metastatic bone disease? It has been suggested, both for clodronate and pamidronate, that patients with humoral hypercalcaemia of malignancy respond poorly to single infusions of drug. To determine this, we reviewed our experience with pamidronate over several years in a total of 160 patients whose characteristics are shown in Table 2. All patients had remained hypercalcaemic following intravenous saline rehydration and received a median dose of 1.0 mg/kg (range 0.25–4.5), the majority (94 of 160) as a single 24-hour infusion. Excluding ten patients who either died early or were lost to follow-up – and in none of whom the serum calcium was increasing – only eight of the 150 remaining patients were still hypercalcaemic after therapy, a success rate of 95%, or 90% ($n = 136$) when calcium is corrected for protein levels. It is worth noting that the

45

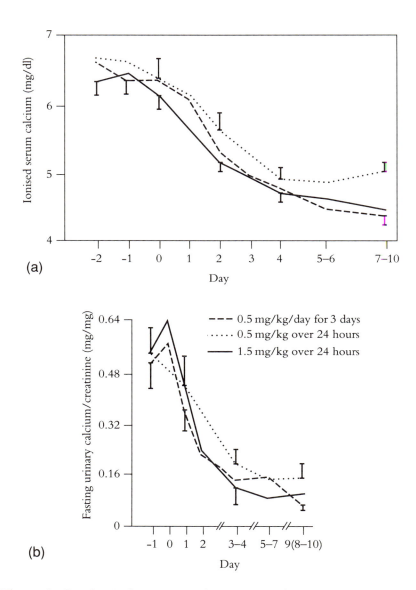

Figure 4 Randomised comparison between pamidronate given either as a daily infusion (0.5 mg/kg) for 3 days or as single infusions of 0.5 mg/kg or 1.5 mg/kg in patients with tumour-induced hypercalcaemia: effect on (a) serum calcium and (b) urinary calcium levels. From Body et al[11], with permission

Table 2   Data on 160 patients (97 female and 63 male: mean age 60 years, range 23–90) with various types of cancer who remained hypercalcaemic after saline rehydration and who then received pamidronate (median dose 1.0 mg/kg, range 0.25–4.5); the majority ($n = 94$) received a single infusion

Tumour site	
Breast	62
Head and neck	36
Lung	21
Other	41
Presence of bone metastases	
Extensive	70
Moderate	30
Doubtful	25
Absent	35

eight patients who failed treatment also showed a significant decrease in serum calcium levels.

The data were then divided into four groups according to tumour site – breast, head and neck, lung and miscellaneous – and according to the presence or absence of bone metastases. At the doses used there were no significant differences in response according to tumour type or extent of bone metastases. A more sensitive parameter of bone resorption, such as the fasting urinary calcium excretion, confirmed these findings.

Side-effects

The only clinically detectable side-effects were a transient drug-induced fever seen in 10–15% of patients, a transient lymphopenia of uncertain clinical relevance, and a decrease in serum phosphate levels due to potent inhibition of bone resorption and recovery of parathyroid function as serum calcium falls.

Combined therapy with other drugs

Bisphosphonate treatment should be combined with intravenous administration of saline; no risk has been demonstrated in giving both at the same time. Combination with calcitonin may be of value in patients with severe life-threatening hypercalcaemia.

Efficacy of a second or third course of pamidronate

In 12 patients who received a second course of pamidronate, the fall in serum calcium was significantly less after the second course than after the first[12]. Renal handling of calcium was similar before each course but urinary hydroxyproline excretion, a marker of bone resorption, was higher before the second course than the first and remained significantly higher after therapy, suggesting that the enhanced bone resorption rate was not inhibited sufficiently by second bisphosphonate administration. We have obtained similar data in 24 patients who received a second course of pamidronate and in ten who received a third course (median dose 1 mg/kg). The fall in serum calcium was significantly less after the second course than after the first, and even less after the third course than after the second, although the mean urinary calcium excretion was not significantly different before each course. It remains to be seen whether increasing the dose for second or third treatments will render patients more susceptible. There are case reports suggesting that this is so, but clearly further studies are required.

CONCLUSIONS

Pamidronate can normalise serum calcium in 90–95% of hypercalcaemic cancer patients. The most effective dose is 60–90 mg (1.0–1.5 mg/kg bodyweight) given as a single infusion over 4–24 hours, or divided into two or three daily 2-hour infusions. At these doses, response is not influenced significantly by tumour type, by the extent of bone metastases or by the type of cancer hypercalcaemia. The drug is well tolerated, and should be combined with intravenous saline and perhaps with calcitonin for patients with severe life-threatening hypercalcaemia. Subsequent infusions seem less efficient than the first, raising the question whether maintenance therapy – by regular infusions or daily oral dosing – or increased doses for second and later courses of treatment provide the best option.

REFERENCES

1. Singer, F. R., Ritch, P. S., Lad, T. E., et al (1991) Treatment of hypercalcaemia of malignancy with intravenous etidronate. *Arch. Intern. Med.*, **151**, 471–6

2. Urwin, G. H., Yates, A. J. P., Gray, R. E. S., et al (1987) Treatment of the hypercalcaemia of malignancy with intravenous clodronate. *Bone*, 8, 543–51

3. Bonjour, J. P., Philippe, J., Guelpa, G., et al (1988) Bone and renal components in hypercalcemia of malignancy and responses to a single infusion of clodronate. *Bone*, **9**, 123–30

4. Dumon, J. C., Magritte, A. and Body, J. J. (1991) Efficacy and safety of the bisphosphonate tiludronate for the treatment of tumor-associated hypercalcemia. *Bone Miner.*, **15**, 257–66

5. Bickerstaff, D. R., O'Doherty, D. P., McCloskey, E. V., et al (1991) Effects of aminobutylidene diphosphonate in hypercalcaemia due to malignancy. *Bone*, **12**, 17–20

6. Harinck, H. I. J., Bijvoet, O. L. M., Plantingh, A. S. T., et al (1987) The role of bone and kidney in tumor-hypercalcemia and its treatment with bisphosphonate and sodium chloride. *Am. J. Med.*, **82**, 1133–42

7. Body, J.-J., Borkowski, A., Cleeren, A., et al (1986) Treatment of malignancy-associated hypercalcaemia with intravenous amino-hydroxypropylidene diphosphonate (APD). *J. Clin. Oncol.*, **4**, 1177–83

8. Thiébaud, D., Jaeger, P., Jacquet, A. F., et al (1986) A single-day treatment of tumor-induced hypercalcaemia by intravenous amino-hydroxypropylidene bisphosphonate. *J. Bone Miner. Res.*, **1**, 555–62

9. Body, J.-J., Pot, M., Borkowski, A., et al (1987) A dose – response study of amino-hydroxypropylidene bisphosphonate in tumor-associated hypercalcemia. *Am. J. Med.*, **82**, 957–63

10. Thiébaud, D., Jaeger, P., Jacquet, A. F., et al (1988) Dose–response in the treatment of hypercalcaemia of malignancy by a single infusion of the bisphosphonate AHPrBP. *J. Clin. Oncol.*, **6**, 762–8

11. Body, J.-J., Magritte, A., Seraj, F., et al (1989) Aminohydroxypropylidene bisphosphonate (APD) treatment for tumor-associated hypercalcemia: a randomized comparison between a 3-day treatment and single 24-hour infusions. *J. Bone Miner. Res.*, **4**, 923–8

12. Thiébaud, D., Jaeger, P. and Burckhardt, P. (1990) Response to retreatment of malignant hypercalcemia with the bisphosphonate AHPrBP (APD): respective role of kidney and bone. *J. Bone Miner. Res.*, **5**, 221–6

13. Body, J.-J. (1991) Treatment of tumour-induced hypercalcaemia with pamidronate – the European experience. In Bijvoet, O. L. M. and Lipton,

A. (eds.) *Osteoclast Inhibition in the Management of Malignancy-related Bone Disorders*, pp. 18–26. (Lewiston, N.Y: Hogrefe and Huber)

14. Coleman, R. E. and Rubens, R. D. (1987) 3(amino-1, 1-hydroxypropyl-idene) bisphosphonate (APD) for hypercalcaemia of breast cancer. *Br. J. Cancer*, **56**, 465–9

15. Ralston, S. H., Alzaid, A. A., Gallacher, S. J., et al (1988) Clinical experience with aminohydroxypropylidene bisphosphonate (APD) in the management of cancer-associated hypercalcaemia. *Q. J. Med.*, **69**, 825–34

16. Cantwell, B. M. J. and Harris, A. L. (1987) Effect of single high dose infusions of aminohydroxypropylidene diphosphonate on hypercalcaemia caused by cancer. *Br. Med. J.*, **294**, 467–9

17. Mannix, K. A., Carmichael, J., Harris, A. L., et al (1989) Single high-dose (45 mg) infusions of aminohydroxypropylidene diphosphonate for severe malignant hypercalcaemia. *Cancer*, **64**, 1358–61

18. Morton, A. R., Cantrill, J. A., Craig, A. E., et al (1988) Single dose versus daily intravenous aminohydroxypropylidene bisphosphonate (APD) for the hypercalcaemia of malignancy. *Br. Med. J.*, **296**, 811–14

19. Sawyer, N., Newstead, C., Drummond, A., et al (1990) Fast (4-h) or slow (24-h) infusions of pamidronate disodium (aminohydroxypropylidene diphosphonate (APD) as single shot treatment of hypercalcaemia. *Bone Miner.*, **9**, 121–8

DISCUSSION

Dr I. Boyle *(Glasgow, UK)* Your data on the distribution of tumour type is very important, bearing in mind the variety and incidence of tumour types in the different studies. Had you not been able to demonstrate that tumour type was unimportant, the regression line might not have been quite so convincing.

Dr Body I agree.

Dr A. Howell *(Manchester, UK)* Your data on resistance to bisphosphonates is also interesting. Can you envisage any mechanism by which this might occur?

Dr Body That is a difficult question but an important one, and probably also for the treatment of normocalcaemic patients with bisphosphonates. We need to know whether patients will become normocalcaemic if the dose is increased; some authors have claimed that, but without real proof.

We are currently trying to investigate this, to determine if some form of resistance to bisphosphonates develops after a certain time.

Professor J. Kanis *(Sheffield, UK)* From time to time, and irrespective of the bisphosphonate used, one sees patients who are resistant, but this is usually very late on in the disease process. I have always interpreted this as being non-osteoclast-mediated bone resorption, and have not seen resistance to bisphosphonates early in the natural history of disease. This is also true for Paget's disease, where several studies of retreatment with bisphosphonates have shown no evidence of resistance. Do you think that resistance relates to the natural history of breast cancer or other neoplastic disease, or is it a special problem of the aminobisphosphonates?

Dr Body Some of our patients were clearly not in the terminal phase of their disease and nevertheless responded poorly. Moreover, some investigators also say that the second course of bisphosphonates is not as efficient as the first in Paget's disease.

Professor Kanis But that is with the aminobisphosphonates. Where a non-nitrogen-containing bisphosphonate has been used, no difference has been found.

Dr Body That is true. Resistance may relate to the disease process, particularly advanced cancer, but there is also the question of the compound itself. Resistance may only apply to some compounds, not others.

4

Treatment of osteolytic bone disease with bisphosphonates

A. Howell

Christie Hospital and Holt Radium Institute, Manchester, UK

SUMMARY

The bisphosphonates, especially clodronate and pamidronate, are active osteolytic agents, and have been shown to be effective in the management of bone metastases in breast and prostate cancer, and myeloma – whether in terms of objective response, rate of appearance of new lesions, reduction in fracture rate, prevention of hypercalcaemia, or reduction in bone pain. This paper reviews the available literature and reaches some tentative conclusions. However, it is particularly difficult to assess response in prostate cancer and myeloma, and different trials have reached different conclusions on the degree of benefit to be derived from a bisphosphonate in respect of the parameters mentioned above. Further study is required to clarify the most appropriate dosing schedules, route of administration, and time to commence therapy.

INTRODUCTION

Antiosteolytic therapy in the treatment of cancer is basically of two kinds (Figure 1):

(1)   Mediator inhibition/cytotoxic effects brought about by endocrine therapy, chemotherapy or radiotherapy; and

(2)   Osteoclast inhibition brought about by calcitonin, mithramycin, gallium nitrate, strontium and the bisphosphonates.

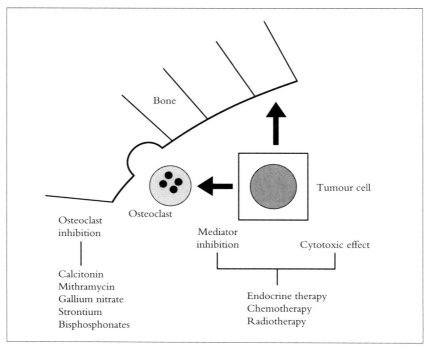

Figure 1 The two basic kinds of osteolytic therapy: mediator inhibition and cytotoxic effects brought about by endocrine therapy; chemotherapy and radiotherapy; and osteoclast inhibition

Because some osteoclast inhibitors are toxic and others exhibit tachyphylaxis, the bisphosphonates have recently come to the fore as potentially useful agents in preventing osteolysis. However, there are some problems in determining the place of bisphosphonates in the treatment of cancer, for example which bisphosphonate to use, which tumour types to treat, how to assess an effect, both objectively and subjectively, and which route of administration to use. And finally, what future studies should be undertaken to establish the place of bisphosphonates in antiosteolytic therapy?

THE BISPHOSPHONATES

Bisphosphonates are chemical analogues of pyrophosphate, a natural inhibitor of crystal nucleation and bone mineralisation. In bisphosphonates the P–O–P bond of pyrophosphate is replaced with a P–C–P bond, which confers a much longer biological half-life and makes the molecule very stable and resistant to enzymic breakdown. The structures of five bisphosphonates are shown in Figure 2, together with the approximate dose (in mg) required to render a patient normocalcaemic after a standard intravenous infusion. The newer bisphosphonates are clearly more potent, but there are insufficient data to include them in this analysis, which will be confined to the first- and second-generation agents etidronate, clodronate and pamidronate.

ASSESSMENT OF EFFICACY

Bisphosphonates have been used mainly for treating bone metastases of breast and prostate cancer, and myeloma. There is little information on

Pyrophosphate $\qquad$ Generic bisphosphonate

$$O = \underset{\underset{OH}{|}}{\overset{\overset{OH}{|}}{P}} - O - \underset{\underset{OH}{|}}{\overset{\overset{OH}{|}}{P}} = O \qquad\qquad O = \underset{\underset{OH}{|}}{\overset{\overset{OH}{|}}{P}} - \underset{\underset{R_2}{|}}{\overset{\overset{R_1}{|}}{C}} - \underset{\underset{OH}{|}}{\overset{\overset{OH}{|}}{P}} = O$$

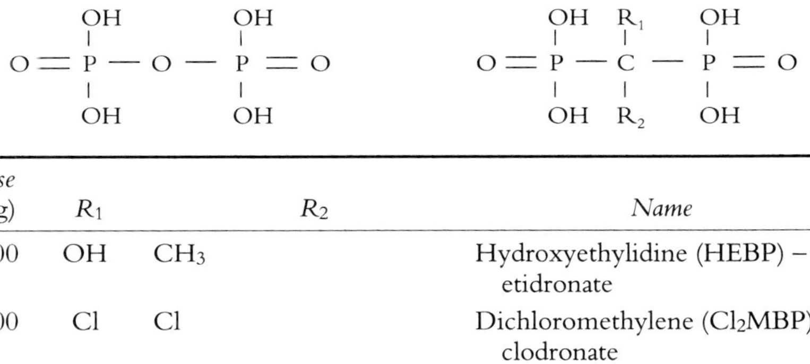

Dose (mg)	R_1	R_2	Name
1500	OH	CH_3	Hydroxyethylidine (HEBP) – etidronate
900	Cl	Cl	Dichloromethylene (Cl_2MBP) – clodronate
60	OH	$(CH_2)_2 - NH_2$	Aminohydroxypropylidine (AHPrBP/APD) – pamidronate
5	OH	$(CH_2)_3 - NH_2$	Aminohydroxybutylidine
1	OH	$(CH_2)_2 - N \overset{\diagup CH_3}{\diagdown (CH_2)_3 - CH_3}$	Hydroxymethylpentenyl-propylidine

Figure 2 Structure of pyrophosphate, a generic bisphosphonate and five bisphosphonates including etidronate, clodronate and pamidronate. The dose (in mg) is that of the individual bisphosphonate required to render a patient normocalcaemic after a standard intravenous infusion

the value of etidronate in patients with bone metastases from breast cancer, and of pamidronate in myeloma. Bone is one of the most difficult sites of metastases for assessment of effect, although five objective measures – response, delay in progression, prevention of fractures, prevention of hypercalcaemia, and survival – and two subjective measures – pain and mobility – have been used.

Objective response

Three studies of pamidronate in breast cancer patients with bone metastases provided the following data (UICC criteria in all cases):

(1)   Morton et al showed four partial remissions (18%) in 22 patients, with a further seven patients (32%) showing stable disease for more than 6 months[1];

(2)   Coleman et al showed four partial remissions (17%) in 24 patients, with a further 11 patients (46%) showing stable disease for more than 3 months[2]; and

(3)   Lipton (personal communication) showed 15 partial remissions (29%) in 52 patients.

Objective response is even more difficult to evaluate in prostate cancer with bone metastases. Clarke et al[3] treated 28 patients with intravenous pamidronate 30 mg every 2 weeks; all patients had end-stage prostatic cancer with bone metastases. Of 11 patients with raised acid phosphatase, six showed a fall, possibly indicative of response. Bone scans were taken at start of treatment and at 6 months; in six of the surviving 12 patients the bone scans showed disease stabilisation, compared with previous progression. These studies provide evidence of objective response to pamidronate used alone in patients with bone metastases.

Rate of appearance of new lesions

Can bisphosphonates reduce the appearance of new bone metastases? In a controlled trial over 12 months comparing clodronate 1600 mg/day plus standard therapy versus placebo plus standard therapy in 34 patients with breast cancer and bone metastases, Elomaa et al[4] showed only three progressions (18%) in the 17 patients on clodronate against 11 progressions (65%) in the 17 patients on placebo, which was a significant difference.

In patients with myeloma there are two controlled trials comparing clodronate with placebo. In a small trial (*n* = 14), Delmas[5] showed no progression of lesions in all seven patients receiving clodronate 1600 mg orally daily over a 6–18 month follow-up period, whereas progression was apparent during this time in five of the seven patients on placebo. In a bigger study[6], clodronate was given to 30 patients intravenously for 7 days and then intramuscularly for 10 days; the cycle was repeated every 4 months. Median follow-up was 24 months. During that time there was progression in only five patients in the treated group (17%), whereas in the control group (*n* = 30: untreated patients not given a placebo) 21 patients (70%) progressed.

Compared to clodronate, etidronate appears ineffective. In a large trial (*n* = 166), Belch et al[7] showed that etidronate, given continuously at a dose of 5 mg/kg bodyweight daily to 92 patients, had a progression rate of 36% (31 of 92 patients), compared to only 27% (20 of 74 patients) in the placebo group.

Reduction in fracture rate

In the same trial[4] referred to above, Elomaa et al noted fewer fractures (*n* =1) in the clodronate arm than in the control arm (*n* = 4). A Dutch study[8] compared pamidronate 300 mg/day continuously in 67 patients with breast cancer and bone metastases with 49 untreated controls, although all patients could receive any other necessary treatment. Median follow-up was 14 months. There were three fractures among patients on pamidronate (4%) but 14 among the controls (29%). A more recent study in patients with breast cancer[9] showed roughly a one-third reduction in vertebral fractures in patients receiving clodronate.

With respect to myeloma, etidronate was again ineffective in reducing fracture rate[7]. Using clodronate, Delmas[5] showed one fracture in the clodronate group (*n* = 7) against four in the placebo group (*n* = 6), while Merlini et al[6] showed three fractures in the clodronate group (*n* = 30) against 15 in the control group (*n* = 30).

Prevention of hypercalcaemia

With clodronate, Elomaa et al[4] saw only one hypercalcaemic episode in 16 treated patients against four in 16 controls. With pamidronate, Cleton et al[8] saw no hypercalcaemic episodes in 70 treated patients against 13 in 53 controls. Similar benefits were seen in patients with myeloma receiving clodronate[6], but once again etidronate was ineffective.

Survival

The data on survival are less promising. In the trial of Elomaa et al[4], 11 of 17 patients receiving clodronate were alive at 2 years compared to only four of 17 on placebo ($p = 0.005$). No other studies have shown a survival advantage, either in breast cancer, prostate cancer or myeloma, whichever bisphosphonate was used. Thus, although they cannot be expected to improve survival, bisphosphonates can be expected to improve quality of life.

Bone pain and mobility

Subjective measures of response, such as relief of bone pain, are very difficult to evaluate. In the three pamidronate studies referred to above, patients ($n = 98$ in total) with advanced breast cancer and osteolytic bone metastases showed a significant reduction in linear analogue pain score. None of these studies was randomised, and the findings may be a placebo effect. However, a randomised study[10], comparing the effect of daily pamidronate 300 mg orally in 76 patients with metastatic breast cancer against controls ($n = 68$), showed a significant reduction in pain scores in the treated group. Each patient was evaluated every 3 months for various events – hypercalcaemia, fracture, bone pain requiring radiotherapy, impairment of mobility – and the scores were added together at each time-point to form a cumulative sum of complications. Pamidronate-treated patients had about 50% fewer events than controls (Figure 3). Specific data on bone pain and impairment of mobility also showed a significant (about 30%) reduction in pain and a significant improvement in mobility in treated patients compared to controls (Figure 4).

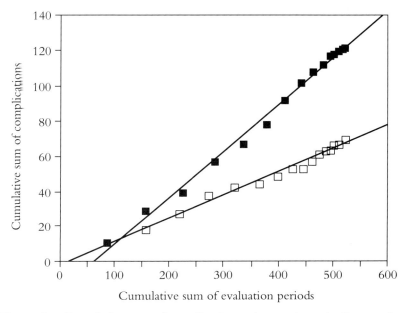

Figure 3 Cumulative sum of complications – hypercalcaemia, fracture, bone pain requiring radiotherapy, impairment of mobility – in patients ($n = 76$) with metastatic breast cancer treated with oral pamidronate 300 mg daily (open squares), compared to untreated controls ($n = 68$: closed squares). (From van Holten-Verzantvoort et al[10], with permission)

With respect to prostate cancer, Adami and Mian[11] treated six patients with clodronate 300 mg intravenously; all were progressing on standard therapies. Compared to seven controls, treated patients showed a reduction in pain score on a linear analogue scale. But clodronate given either *orally* ($n = 11$) or *intramuscularly* ($n = 12$) in another group of patients over 4 weeks had no effect on pain.

In another study by the same authors[11], patients with various different cancers were randomised to one of three groups to receive either oral clodronate 1200 mg daily for 2 weeks; intravenous clodronate 300 mg intravenously over 2 weeks; or intravenous clodronate as above followed by oral clodronate 1200 mg/day. Oral clodronate alone had little effect on pain scores, whereas clodronate given intravenously over a 2-week period reduced pain scores significantly. When oral clodronate was given following intravenous infusion, again there was a significant difference

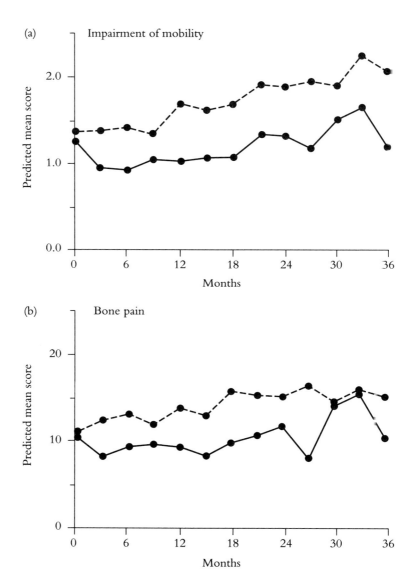

Figure 4 Predicted mean scores over time for (a) impairment of mobility and (b) bone pain in patients (*n* = 76) with metastatic breast cancer treated with oral pamidronate 300 mg daily (●——●), compared to untreated controls (*n* = 68, ●---●). (From van Holten-Verzantvoort et al[11], with permission)

Table 1 Magnitude of effect of clodronate and pamidronate on objective and subjective parameters of response in breast (B) and prostate (P) cancer and in myeloma (M). The figures represent the results of individual trials

Parameter of response	Improvement with clodronate (%)	Improvement with pamidronate (%)
Objective response		
Partial response	—	17–29 (B)
Stable disease	—	21–32 (B and P)
Delay in appearance of new lesions	73 (B)	—
	76	—
Prevention of fractures	75 (B)	79 (B)
	75 (M)	—
	80 (M)	—
Prevention of hypercalcaemia	75 (B)	100 (B)
	66 (M)	—
Survival	64 (B)	n.s. (B)
	n.s. (B)	
	n.s. (P)	
Pain	46 (P)	66 (B)
	70 (P)	6 (B)
	50 (P)	0 (B)
	80 (M)	33 (B)

($p < 0.005$) between those patients receiving such maintenance therapy and those who did not receive it. These are the most clear-cut data showing a beneficial effect of bisphosphonates on pain from any sort of cancer.

There are four other studies relating to control of bone pain in patients with prostate cancer. Smith[12] showed etidronate to be ineffective in a small placebo-controlled trial. Clarke et al[3] gave pamidronate 30 mg intravenously every 2 weeks to 26 patients, and showed that the proportion free of pain increased from 31% to 57% over a 6-month period, suggesting that pamidronate was effective. Kylmälä et al[13] compared 40 patients given oral clodronate (3200 mg daily for 1 month, then 1600 mg daily) with a placebo group ($n = 41$). After 1 year's follow-up, 33 patients (82%) in the treated group were pain free, compared to only ten (24%) in the placebo group.

With respect to bone pain in myeloma, etidronate was again ineffec-tive[7], but clodronate – given intravenously for 7 days then intramuscularly for 10 days – produced a significant reduction in bone pain, with only four of 30 treated patients experiencing pain compared to 20 of 30 controls.

SUMMARY AND CONCLUSIONS

The effect of clodronate and pamidronate on objective response, delay in progression, reduction in fractures, prevention of hypercalcaemia, survival, and pain and mobility suggests that bisphosphonates have a marked effect on various objective and subjective estimates of response, achieving a 70% reduction in some of the parameters (Table 1).

Both clodronate and pamidronate are active osteolytic agents, produc-ing objective and subjective responses. The most appropriate dosing schedules and optimal route of administration need further clarification. The hypothesis – that treatment earlier in the course of disease is more effective – needs to be tested, and trials are currently under way in which a bisphosphonate is given as adjuvant therapy after surgery for breast cancer, and at first relapse in patients without bone disease but who may ultimately develop it, to see whether the onset of bone disease can be prevented. Finally, the testing of new and more active bisphosphonates should continue.

REFERENCES

1. Morton, A. R., Cantrill, J. A., Pillai, G. V., et al (1988) Sclerosis of lytic bone metastases after disodium aminohydroxypropylidene bisphosphonate (APD) in patients with breast carcinoma. *Br. Med. J.*, **297**, 772–3
2. Coleman, R. E., Woll, P. J., Miles, M., et al (1988) Treatment of bone metastases from breast cancer with 3-amino-1-hydroxypropylidene-1,1-bisphosphonate (APD). *Br. J. Cancer*, **58**, 621–5
3. Clarke, N.W., Holbrook, I. B., McClure, J., et al (1991) Osteoclast inhibition by pamidronate in metastatic prostate cancer: a preliminary study. *Br. J. Cancer*, **63**, 420–3
4. Elomaa, I., Blomqvist, C., Porkka, L., et al (1985) Diphosphonates for osteolytic metastases. *Lancet*, **i**, 1155–6
5. Delmas, P. D. (1991) The use of clodronate in multiple myeloma. *Bone*, **12** (Suppl. 1), 531–4

6. Merlini, G., Parrinello, G. A., Piccinini, L., et al (1990) Long-term effects of parenteral dichloromethylene bisphosphonate (CL2MPB) on bone disease of myeloma patients treated with chemotherapy. *Hematol. Oncol.*, **8**, 23–30

7. Belch, A. R., Bergsagel, D. E., Wilson, K., et al (1991) Effect of daily etidronate on the osteolysis of multiple myeloma. *J. Clin. Oncol.*, **9**, 1397–1402

8. Cleton, F. J., van Holten-Verzantvoort, A. T. and Bijvoet, O. L. (1989) Effect of long-term bisphosphonate treatment on morbidity due to bone metastases in breast cancer patients. *Recent Results Cancer Res.*, **116**, 73–8

9. Paterson, A. H., Ernst, D. S., Powles, T., et al (1991) Treatment of skeletal disease in breast cancer with clodronate. *Bone*, **12** (Suppl. 1), 525–30

10. van Holten-Verzantvoort, A. T., Zwinderman, A. H., Aaronson, N. K., et al (1991) The effect of supportive pamidronate treatment on aspects of quality of life of patients with advanced breast cancer. *Eur. J. Cancer*, **27**, 544–9

11. Adami, S. and Mian, M. (1989) Clodronate therapy of metastatic bone disease in patients with prostate carcinoma. *Recent Results Cancer Res.*, **116**, 67–72

12. Smith, J. A. (1989) Palliation of painful bone metastases from prostate cancer using sodium etidronate: results of a randomised, prospective double-blind, placebo-controlled study. *J. Urol.*, **141**, 85–7

13. Kylmälä, T., Tammela, T., Elomaa, I., et al (1991) The effect of clodronate on metastatic bone pain in prostate cancer. 22nd European Symposium on Calcified Tissue, March 1991, Vienna. *Tissue Int.*, **48** (Suppl.), A38. (Abst.)

5

Non-oncological uses of bisphosphonates

D. Heath

Department of Medicine, Queen Elizabeth Hospital,
Birmingham, UK

SUMMARY

Bisphosphonates are effective in Paget's disease of bone, in osteoporosis – both in the treatment of established disease and as preventive therapy – and in heterotopic calcification. With respect to Paget's disease, doubts remain concerning which bisphosphonate should be used, which patients should be treated, how long treatment should last and how it should be monitored. There is also concern that bisphosphonates in high doses may harm bone formation.

INTRODUCTION

Bisphosphonates are best known in the management of hypercalcaemia of malignancy and osteolytic bone metastases. However, it has recently become clear that they are also effective in other non-oncological disorders such as Paget's disease of bone, osteoporosis, and heterotopic calcification.

BISPHOSPHONATES IN PAGET'S DISEASE

Bisphosphonates are the treatment of choice for Paget's disease of bone, whatever criteria are used to assess efficacy. Debate now revolves around which biphosphonate should be used, who should be treated, how long treatment should last, and how it should be monitored. This paper outlines the author's current practice.

Which bisphosphonate should be used?

The available drugs are etidronate, pamidronate and clodronate, although only etidronate is *licensed* for treatment of Paget's disease. Etidronate and clodronate are both available as oral and intravenous formulations, but in the UK pamidronate is currently available only as an intravenous formulation.

Oral therapy has the great advantage of enabling patients to be treated outside hospital, but it also has a major disadvantage: the bisphosphonates show extremely poor oral absorption (about 4%), and this is reduced even further if taken with food or a calcium preparation. A bisphosphonate has to be taken on an empty stomach – 2 hours after a meal and 2 hours before the next meal – and some patients find this confusing.

Intravenous therapy has the advantage of accurate dosing and greater potency but requires regular visits to the hospital. Clinicians need to decide on the most appropriate way to treat their patients, given the individual circumstances of each.

Who should be treated?

Uncontroversial indications are symptomatic bone pain not controlled by simple analgesics, and cord compression. When caused by Paget's disease, cord compression responds extremely well to medical treatment, the results of which equate with surgical treatment. Other patients with Paget's disease, who do not fall within these treatment criteria, can be treated if deemed appropriate. At one extreme, some doctors believe that every patient with Paget's disease should be treated; at the other are doctors who accept only the two major indications specified above. It remains to be seen whether bisphosphonates will prevent or reduce the incidence of fractures, deformity or hearing loss.

How long should treatment last?

There are two schools of thought. The first maintains that patients should be treated until their symptoms are well controlled; the second, that treatment should continue until all biochemical markers of the disease have returned to the normal range. Some doctors who take the latter view claim that such patients are cured, but the evidence for that remains uncertain.

How should treatment be monitored?

There are various ways to monitor treatment: serum alkaline phosphatase, urinary hydroxyproline or pyridinum cross-links, bone scans, X-rays or even bone biopsies. Much depends on the aims of treatment. If the doctor is primarily concerned with the relief of pain, it can be argued that none of these parameters need to be measured. If total biochemical remission is the goal, then several such parameters will need to be monitored.

Summary

My own practice is only to treat patients who are symptomatic – patients whose pain cannot be controlled with simple analgesics. At present I use oral etidronate 400 mg/day on an outpatient basis, and stop treatment at 3 months if there is no improvement in pain, or at 9 months if the patient responds. The reason for stopping treatment at 9 months is the very real concern that continued bisphosphonate therapy, particularly at higher doses, may cause fractures. I use the serum alkaline phosphatase as the only marker of biochemical control.

BISPHOSPHONATES IN OSTEOPOROSIS

In osteoporosis, bisphosphonates can be used both in the treatment of established disease and as preventive therapy. In three controlled clinical trials of the efficacy of etidronate and calcium[1-3], etidronate was given for 2 weeks every 3 months, and calcium supplements for the other 11 weeks, before repeating the cycle. In another controlled trial[4], tiludronate was given continuously for 6 months, then discontinued for a further 6 months; at the end of the year beneficial effects could still be seen. Etidronate is now licensed in the UK for the treatment of established osteoporosis. To my knowledge there are, as yet, no published data available on the use of bisphosphonates in the *prevention* of osteoporosis.

We have undertaken an open, uncontrolled study to investigate the effects of etidronate in patients with established osteoporosis. After 12 months' treatment, the density of the spinal bone, as measured by DEXA, had increased by 5.9% and that at the hip by 1.6%. Similar results have been reported in other studies with etidronate. We are also undertaking a controlled study in women who do not wish to consider hormone replacement therapy. At 1 year, control patients are showing the expected mean small losses in bone mass at the spine (−1.52%) and the hip (−2.53%), whereas cyclical etidronate has essentially prevented bone loss at the hip (−0.12%) and has increased bone mass in the spine (+1.82%). Our experience suggests that the bisphosphonates will be of value in preventing loss of bone mass, both in established osteoporosis and as a prophylactic treatment. They are not, in any sense, an alternative to hormone replacement therapy, certainly in the prevention of osteoporosis, because there are many other advantages of hormone replacement therapy over and above its benefits on the skeleton. Nevertheless, a significant number of women do not want (or cannot have) hormone replacement therapy, and in this population a bisphosphonate may well be the drug of choice.

BISPHOSPHONATES IN HETEROTOPIC CALCIFICATION

Some studies have suggested that bisphosphonates may prevent heterotopic calcification in patients undergoing hip replacement. Some doctors, especially in the United States, have advocated their use as routine prophylaxis, but this seems excessive. However, if a hip replacement has been plagued by heterotopic calcification, it seems reasonable to prescribe a bisphosphonate prior to a subsequent replacement in order to prevent or reduce the problem.

DO BISPHOSPHONATES HARM BONE?

Bisphosphonates are taken up into bone and can remain there for many months. Early studies which used high-dose etidronate caused a higher incidence of fractures. All bisphosphonates, if used at a sufficiently high dose, will reduce bone formation, and this risk is probably greater with etidronate. However, at the dose recommended for treatment of Paget's disease, the available studies suggest that etidronate − used for a limited period of time − reduces the fracture rate.

In osteoporosis there are as yet no long-term data, and detailed post-marketing surveillance is required. To date, studies in osteoporosis have shown that, whatever the bisphosphonates may do to bone formation, bone mass is increased, suggesting benefit to patients.

REFERENCES

1. Storm, T., Tharnsborg, G., Steiniche, T., et al (1990) Effect of intermittent cyclical etidronate therapy on bone mass and fracture rate in postmenopausal osteoporosis. *N. Engl. J. Med.*, **322**, 1265–71
2. Watts, N. B., Harris, S. T., Genant, H. K., et al (1990) Intermittent cyclical etidronate treatment of postmenopausal osteoporosis. *N. Engl. J. Med.*, **323**, 73–9
3. Miller, P. D., Neal, B. J., McIntyre, D. O., et al (1991) Effect of cyclical therapy with phosphorus and etidronate on axial bone mineral density in postmenopausal osteoporotic women. *Osteoporosis Int.*, **1**, 171–6
4. Reginster, J. Y., Lecart, M. P., Deroisy, R., et al (1989) Prevention of postmenopausal bone loss by tiludronate. *Lancet*, **ii**, 1469–71

DISCUSSION

Professor R. D. Rubens *(London, UK)* Why are antiosteoclastic agents effective in osteoporosis?

Dr Heath I believe that they reduce bone resorption more than they inhibit bone formation, establishing a positive balance.

Professor Rubens But is osteoporosis not primarily a disease of the protein structure of the bone, rather than a fault in its calcification?

Dr Heath Certainly some of the severe forms of osteoporosis, particularly in young people, are caused by abnormal collagen and have nothing to do with abnormalities of calcification. But even so, if you can reduce overall bone loss, that must be beneficial.

Dr R. Coleman *(Sheffield, UK)* In malignancy, the duration of action of a single dose of a bisphosphonate is several weeks. I understand that in Paget's disease it can be months or even years. Can you explain why there should be such a difference?

Dr Heath   I am not sure that I can. It is said that at least one-third of patients with Paget's disease remain in long-term remission after 5–9 months of treatment, very similar to the experience with calcitonin. It may be that the disease mechanism is switched off in a percentage of patients, as in the management of Graves' disease, but I have no firm information.

6

Panel discussion

Dr L. Boyle *(Glasgow, UK)*   The long natural history of many patients with breast cancer provides an excellent opportunity for clinical intervention, with an impact both on morbidity and mortality. However, no single biochemical parameter is available to distinguish between disease progression and therapeutic response. Can Dr Coleman comment on whether osteotropism is a chemotactic phenomenon in breast and prostatic cancer, or is there a more mundane mechanical or anatomical explanation?

Dr R Coleman *(Sheffield, UK)*   There are vascular channels – described many years ago – that may explain why tumour cells metastasise preferentially to the spine. This seems more convincing for prostate than for breast cancer. What surprises me is that patients can live for years with skeletal metastases which do not themselves metastasise, as is usually the case with metastases in other sites.

Professor R. D. Rubens *(London, UK)*   Professor Kanis used the term coupling on several occasions. What is the coupling signal between osteoblasts and osteoclasts?

Dr Boyle   The chemical message that activates osteoblast precursors following bone resorption is not known, but as osteoclasts erode bone they release substances from the bone matrix. These substances – bone morphogenetic protein or growth factors – stimulate the maturity of pre-osteoblasts in what has been called the cytokine soup. My question is this: how is it that in prostatic cancer new bone can be formed on trabeculae without resorption?

Dr J.-J. Body *(Brussels, Belgium)*   Prostatic cancer cells can synthesise growth factors for osteoblasts, some of which resemble fibroblast growth factor. This raises the question whether it is logical to prescribe anti-osteoclastic drugs in the knowledge that factors synthesised by the tumours are acting directly on osteoblasts.

Professor Rubens   But in osteosclerotic bone disease – particularly in prostatic cancer – CT scans clearly show islands of lytic disease as well, don't they?

Dr Body   That may be due to coupling in bone turnover, with messages going from the osteoblasts to the osteoclasts. I must however say that there is some evidence suggesting activation of osteoclasts by prostate cancer cells.

Dr A. Howell *(Manchester, UK)*   It can be shown *in vitro* that breast tumour cells produce factors that stimulate both osteoblasts *and* osteoclasts. The favoured explanation for the effect of pamidronate in bone disease is that it switches off the osteoclast, although tumour still produces osteoblast stimulating factors, which explains the resclerosis.

Dr Body   Breast cancer cells can certainly secrete osteoblast activating factors such as TGF-β, but they can also secrete factors that inhibit the growth of osteoblasts: we have data to that effect.

Dr Howell   There are similar data for myelomatosis.

Mr S. B. Desai *(Scunthorpe, UK)*   Patients with breast cancer can survive 15–20 years without metastases. Then the husband dies or some other stress arises, and suddenly there are widespread metastases. What is the natural history of these cells, which must have escaped at the time of primary treatment? Have they lain dormant for 15–20 years? How do they survive in the bone marrow?

Dr Coleman   I do not know the answer to that, though the phenomenon is well recognised. I assume that these cells enter a resting phase until certain changes in immunological status reawaken them. There are data to suggest that life events can help to precipitate a recurrence, and that must almost certainly have an immunological basis.

Professor Rubens   Dr Coleman, you have investigated biochemical parameters which appear to predict for potential early response in bone. Do you routinely use these parameters when monitoring patients under treatment for metastatic bone disease?

Dr Coleman   Certainly this is an area that I want to develop, but I am a little disappointed that – with all the excitement about new treatments for bone metastases – nobody has grasped the nettle of assessment parameters. They need to be addressed soon, both for symptom assessment and biochemical control.

Professor Rubens   Dr Howell, have you any comments on the use of biochemical parameters for assessing response?

Dr Howell   No, but I would like to mention the exciting studies just commenced in Denmark using bisphosphonates as preventive therapy after mastectomy. Patients are receiving tamoxifen plus either pamidronate or placebo, and I know that Dr Trevor Powles (Royal Marsden Hospital, UK) is studying the prevention of bone metastases in this way. Over the next 2–3 years we are likely to see whether bisphosphonates are important preventive agents. There are other trials investigating various aspects of advanced disease which could determine the absolute place of bisphosphonates in the treatment of advanced malignant disease in bone.

Professor Rubens   Dr Boyle, have you any thoughts on the biochemical assessment of response in bone?

Dr Boyle   Hydroxyproline is commonly used as a measure of resorption, but it is very imprecise, and is altered by dietary constituents even when early morning fasting samples are taken. Collagen cross-links may well give an earlier indication of resorption.

Professor Rubens   It seems to me that biochemical assessment of bone response is of considerable importance, particularly for those patients receiving treatment which they find unpleasant. Knowing, a month or so after starting treatment, that they are likely to respond can be encouraging. Knowing that they are not likely to respond provides an opportunity to stop unpleasant treatment and reconsider.

Dr Body   Biochemical markers should be used more often, especially now that new markers of bone formation and resorption are available. Moreover, tumour markers such as CA15-3 are also insufficiently used in the evaluation of patients.

Professor Rubens   Dr Howell, I believe that you have studied other markers?

Dr Howell   Yes. We undertook a study using pamidronate as sole therapy in patients with advanced disease, and showed that some patients had resclerosis while others had stabilisation of disease for at least 6 months. In a proportion of patients the tumour markers declined, whereas in others they remained stable: this provided an early indication of effect. In the same study we evaluated the effect of pamidronate on bone pain using a linear analogue scale, and found that pain was reduced by about 50% over 12–16 weeks. Dr Coleman uses a much broader estimation of pain – the so-called pain score – and I wonder whether this should be used in future studies?

Dr Coleman   It is worth looking at again prospectively, but there are others, for example the Oswestry symptom score, which is a pain score originally designed for young fit people with back pain. It is very well structured and has been validated in that situation.

Dr Howell   About 50% of patients with advanced bone cancer are helped by a bisphosphonate, while the other 50% may well not need one at all, because in those cases the mechanism of osteolysis may not be osteoclast-mediated, though I have no data to support that view. An interesting study in Newcastle compared patients receiving the aromatase inhibitor aminoglutethimide plus pamidronate 30 mg by infusion every 3 weeks with patients receiving aminoglutethimide only, and found no differences in fracture rate, incidence of hypercalcaemia, or pain score. This suggests that the same patients respond to both endocrine and bisphosphonate therapy, and that patients with less aggressive, more long-term bone disease respond to bisphosphonates, rather than those with more aggressive disease.

Professor Rubens   Dr Cantwell, is your trial sufficiently powerful at this stage to provide conclusive information? And secondly, if it is not showing beneficial effects attributable to the bisphosphonate, is it not at variance with other reports?

Dr B. M. J. Cantwell *(Newcastle, UK)*   To date, approximately 93 patients have been enrolled into the study. Analyses undertaken at 30 patients and 60 patients have failed to reveal any benefit for the combination of bisphosphonate with aminoglutethimide and low-dose hydrocortisone. The explanation is unclear: perhaps these agents might best be used sequentially rather than together, or perhaps the dose of bisphosphonate – 30 mg every 3 weeks – is insufficient to show an effect.

Dr J. Ford *(Basle, Switzerland)*   The tropism of breast cancer metastases to certain organs is very interesting. Is there any evidence to show that breast cancer cells in bone metastases produce factors that stimulate osteoclasts, whereas similar cells in skin metastases do not?

Dr Body   I know of no specific data. However, it is known that estrogen receptor-positive breast tumours metastasise to bone about three times more often than estrogen receptor-negative tumours, so perhaps there is a clue here.

Dr Coleman   Nigel Bundred (Withington Hospital, Manchester) has provided interesting data on expression of parathyroid hormone related protein (PTHrP) in breast cancer. This protein is present in about 30% of cases of primary breast cancer, but in patients who develop bone metastases the figure rises to around 60%; in those with overwhelming lytic disease and hypercalcaemia the figure is about 80–90%. So PTHrP seems a more powerful predictor for bone metastases than estrogen receptor status.

Professor Rubens   There is a suspicion that bisphosphonates may mask the progression of cancer, with adverse consequences for clinical management. Dr Coleman, I believe your study suggested a higher than expected risk of spinal cord compression. Do bisphosphonates predispose to progression of disease outside the skeleton?

Dr Coleman   The data are insufficient to draw any firm conclusion. The unpublished clodronate studies suggest an increased risk of spinal cord compression. Any doubts in this area could be resolved by serial MRI scanning of the spine, to look at what is happening to the soft tissue component of a bone metastasis while healing is taking place in response to bisphosphonate therapy.

Dr Howell   We saw no such problems in our study, but Alan Lipton's study in patients with prostate cancer had one or two cases of cord compression. So far as I am aware, this problem has not emerged from the randomised Dutch studies or from the clodronate studies.

Professor Rubens   And in any event these patients are at high risk of developing this complication. Finally, what about gallium nitrate as an osteoclast inhibitor?

Dr Howell   Gallium nitrate certainly inhibits osteoclast activity and resolves hypercalcaemia, but it has substantial toxicity, no apparent advantages over a bisphosphonate, and treatment takes 5 days. A bisphosphonate requires a short infusion, which is a dramatic advance in the treatment of hypercalcaemia.

Dr G. P. Deutsch *(Brighton, UK)*   The Danes are undertaking an adjuvant study with bisphosphonates. Will this have a survival advantage, and if so by what mechanism?

Dr Howell   Certain cells within the bone marrow are not adherent to bone but separated from it. Adjuvant therapy with a bisphosphonate may stop these cells invading bone and producing metastases. Some 70% of patients have bone metastases at death, a significant number – about 20% – with bone metastases only. If a bisphosphonate could inhibit that 20%.... The results of the Danish trial and of another undertaken by Trevor Powles may well show some advantages in the future.

Index